C000166116

Ayurvedic Diet

A Beginner's 4-Week Step-by-Step Guide to
Healing and Weight Loss With Curated Recipes

Copyright © 2020 Bruce Ackerberg
All rights reserved. No portion of this book may be reproduced in any form without
permission from the publisher, except as permitted by U.S. copyright law.

Disclaimer

By reading this disclaimer, you are accepting the terms of the disclaimer in full. If you disagree with this disclaimer, please do not read the book. The content in this book is provided for informational and educational purposes only.

This book is not intended to be a substitute for the original work of this diet plan. At most, this book is intended to be a beginner's supplement to the original work for this diet plan and never acts as a direct substitute. This book is an overview, review, and commentary on the facts of that diet plan.

All product names, diet plans, or names used in this book are for identification purposes only and are property of their respective owners. The use of these names does not imply endorsement. All other trademarks cited herein are the property of their respective owners.

None of the information in this book should be accepted as an independent medical or other professional advice.

The information in the books has been compiled from various sources that are deemed reliable. It has been analyzed and summarized to the best of the Author's ability, knowledge, and belief. However, the Author cannot guarantee the accuracy and thus should not be held liable for any errors.

You acknowledge and agree that the Author of

this book will not be held liable for any damages, costs, expenses, resulting from the application of the information in this book, whether directly or indirectly. You acknowledge and agree that you assume all risk and responsibility for any action you undertake in response to the information in this book. You acknowledge and agree that by continuing to read this book, you will (where applicable, appropriate, or necessary) consult a qualified medical professional on this information. The information in this book is not intended to be any sort of medical advice and should not be used in lieu of any medical advice by a licensed and qualified medical professional. Always seek the advice of your physician or another qualified health provider with any issues or questions you might have regarding any sort of medical condition. Do not ever disregard any qualified professional medical advice or delay seeking that advice because of anything you have read in this book.

Table of Contents

Chapter 1: Introduction

Staying healthy is the top priority for almost everyone, and our day-to-day decisions will decide how successful we are in staying healthy. Not everything is in our hands, but our health habits and behaviors often can change the way we are healthy or unhealthy.

Our diet and exercise are two areas in which we have the most control. These can have a major impact on overall health and can be key factors for disease prevention and other complications later in life. Protection measures such as diet and exercise can also support your budget.

A well-balanced diet provides you with all the energy you need for growing and recovering nutrients, helping you stay strong and healthy, and helping you avoid diet-related diseases such as cancers and heart conditions. Eating healthy and having an active balanced diet can also help you keep your weight healthy.

Too important to ignore is the connection between good nutrition and healthy weight, reduced risk of chronic disease, and overall health. You'll be on the way to having the nutrients that the body requires to remain balanced, productive, and strong by taking action to eat healthily. Just like physical activity, it can go a long way to make small changes in your diet, and it is easier than you think!

Non-Western approaches to wellness, from massage and yoga to acupuncture and aromatherapy, have become increasingly popular. There has also been increased interest in the diet for prevention and therapy and learning of the food habits of healthier people around the world. The Ayurvedic diet is one in particular.

The Ayurvedic diet has been based on the tenets of Ayurvedic medicine for a thousand years. The aim is to achieve better synergy and improve the health of the body and mind, integrating different energies within the body.

Would you like to protect yourself from all diseases? Or do you have any chronic disease and want to rid yourself of it naturally and without any medicine? If so, this Ayurvedic diet plan will assist you in preventing and curing certain diseases. This guide will take you on a healthy lifestyle journey through the Ayurvedic diet.

In this guide you will discover...

- The basics of the Ayurvedic diet

- What is dosha and how to identify your dosha

- The health benefits of practicing the Ayurvedic diet

- Four weeks of trusted recipes and a meal plan that will help you lose weight and improve your health condition.

Take control today and start your journey of weight loss and healthy living with the Ayurvedic diet.

Chapter 2: What is the Ayurvedic Diet?

Ayurveda is an ancient Hindu holistic approach to health that serves as a system of the all-embracing mental, physical, and Spiritual Care. Ayurveda means "The wisdom for long life." The tradition teaches that, based on the 'Tri-Dosha' theory, everyone consists of five elements: fire, air, water, earth, space. Under the principles of Ayurveda, fire, air, and water elements are associated with Pitta, Vata, and Kapha, while earth and space elements are constant.

You eat mainly whole or minimally processed foods when you adopt the Ayurvedic diet and observe mindful eating rituals.

You will incorporate many different practices into your eating routine if you follow an Ayurvedic diet. These activities allow you to take advantage of different food qualities.

One of the main features of an Ayurvedic diet is that you eat according to your predominant type of Constitution or **dosha**. Your dosha can be considered your most prominent strength.

Three Ayurvedic doshas come from five different elements: space, air, fire, water, and earth. Each factor has different attributes or qualities.

Vata: Vatas are often characterized as innovative, intense, or expressive (space and air). The features are dry, light, cold, and rough. Pitta (fire and water): often identified as smart, happy, and motivated, pittas. Sharp, hot, liquid, and mobile are some of its attributes.

Kapha (earth and water): Kaphas are often described as being calm, affectionate, or lethargic. Moist, strong, flexible, and static are some of its attributes.

People are believed to be born with doshas. Usually, there are one or two dominant doshas that determine our physical, mental, and emotional properties. For example, the dominant dosha is why one person can't tolerate humidity or oily foods, while another person may react.

Each of the doshas in Ayurveda thrives on a specific diet, lifestyle, and exercise regime. Dosha imbalance can be corrected by modifying diet and lifestyle factors. An imbalance may lead to illness if left unchecked. An ayurvedic practitioner can evaluate a person through a personal and family history and a physical examination.

The Coloration of your Tongue May signifies a Dosha Imbalance.

A person's color of the tongue can indicate an imbalance of dosha. A white tongue coating, for example, can suggest an accumulation of mucus and imbalance in Kapha Dosha.

Each dosha is often connected to a different pulse type. An ayurvedic practitioner evaluates six pulse points (three surface pulses and three deep pulses) on each wrist.

In an ayurvedic assessment, the eyes and fingernails are also observed. If the white color of the eyes is reddish, and the nails are moderate pink, it signifies the pitta dosha.

You may find that after reading descriptions of each dosha, one sounds more like the qualities that you incarnate. Many people have two powerful doshas.

Those who practice ayurvedic lifestyle believe that all three doshas are incarnated by us. Your prominent dosha determines the style of your food.

How to Identify your dosha

There are three central metabolic types or bodily humor in Ayurveda, the former Indian health science system that comprise the constitution of a person.

These are called "doshas" and are the basic forces behind the physical, mental, and emotional structure of a person. The three doshas are known as 'Vata,' 'Pitta,' and 'Kapha.' Ayurveda diets offer ways to achieve healthy, fulfilled lives. Read the questions below to decide your predominant Dosha.

How to identify your Dosha?

Choose the answer for each category that applies most to you. If there is more than one answer, select the one that suits best. For personality and mental characteristics, respond as you felt and acted most of your life.

Physical Characteristics

1. Your height is:

Taller or shorter than average

Average

Tall and large

2. Your body frame is:

Slim and light, with thin muscles

Moderate and symmetrical, with well-developed muscles

Large and ample, with strong muscles

3. Your weight is:

Below average

Average

Above average

4. Regarding your weight changes, you find it:
Hard to gain weight
Easy to maintain weight
Hard to lose weight

5. Your skin texture is:
Dry, rough, and thin; prone to goosebumps
Warm and oily; easily irritated or inflamed
Cool, clammy, and thick

6. Your eyes are:
Small, dry, and active
Piercing; sensitive to light
Large and soft

7. Your hair is:
Dry and brittle; easily knotted
Medium texture and oily; tendency toward thinning or graying
Thick and oily; abundant

8. Your teeth are:
Crooked or protruding; receding gums
Moderately sized, with a tendency toward yellowing; red or bleeding gums
White, strong, and well-formed; hearty gums

9. Your nails are:
Dry, rough, and brittle; they break easily
Soft, pink, flexible, and lustrous
Thick, smooth, shiny, and hard

10. Your joints are:
Prominent; they crack easily
Medium, loose, and flexible
Large and well-padded

11. Your hands are:
Thin; long fingers with prominent knuckles
Medium; warm, pink, and soft
Large and thick; smooth knuckles
12. Your body temperature runs:
Cold, especially your hands and feet; you have poor circulation
Higher than average; you tend to "run hot"
Cool; clammy
13. Your urine tends to be:
Scanty, clear
Abundant, yellow
A moderate amount, concentrated color
14. When you get sick, it's usually in the form of:
Pain and inflammation
Fever and skin irritations, such as cold sores
Congestion
15. When it comes to weather, you dislike:
Cold, dryness, wind; you prefer warm weather
Heat, blazing sunshine, fire; you prefer cool, well-ventilated areas
Cool and damp weather; although you can tolerate many different climates, you prefer it not to be cool and damp.
Personality Traits
16. Your speech tends to be:
Fast and frequent
Sharp and cutting
Slow and melodious
17. In general, you are mostly:

Active, busy, hustling, changeable, or nervous
Ambitious, motivated, competitive, and witty
Calm, content, conservative, and rarely irritated
18. At your best, you are:
Adaptable, creative, spiritual, and imaginative; an abstract thinker
Courageous, intelligent, focused, and efficient; a perfectionist
Loving, trustworthy, caring, calm, and patient; a kind soul
19. At your worst, you are:
Fearful and nervous
Angry and critical
Overly attached and lazy
Food and Activity
20. When it comes to activity, you like:
To be active and on the go; it's hard for you to sit still
Physical activities with a purpose; competitive pursuits
Leisurely activities; sitting around
21. You walk:
Quickly, often looking at the ground
Purposefully, with focus and attention
Slowly and leisurely
22. Your appetite:
Varies daily; you sometimes forget to eat
Is regular; you never skip a meal
Is steady; you like eating but can skip meals easily
23. You tend to eat and digest:

Quickly

Moderately

Slowly

24. When your digestion is out of whack, you get:

Gassy or constipated

Ulcers and heartburn

Lethargic and overweight

25. Your favorite foods are:

Salty, crunchy, or cold; carbonated or caffeinated drinks

Spicy, sour, or bitter; BBQ sauce, meat, pickles, fried food

Creamy, sweet, heavy, or soft

26. Your stamina is:

Quickly depleted; you get worn out easily

Fairly strong; you can handle various physical activities

Good; you have a steady energy level

27. Your sleeping habits are:

Light; you have difficulty falling and staying asleep

Consistent; you sleep well for an average amount of time

Deep; you sleep long and sound, and have difficulty waking up

Mind and Emotions

28. Your moods:

Change quickly

Change slowly

Are mostly steady

29. When under stress, you become:
Excited, anxious, worried, and fearful
Angry, critical, demanding, and aggressive
Withdrawn, depressed, and reclusive
30. When it comes to making a decision:
You have lots of ideas and change your mind easily
You gather facts before forming an opinion
You are stubborn; you make up your mind quickly and don't change your mind often
31. Your attention span is:
Short
Detail-oriented and attentive
On the "big picture"; you can focus for long periods
32. Your memory is:
Short; you learn quickly and forget quickly
Generally good
Good for the long-term, though you learn slowly
33. When it comes to projects, you are:
Good at getting things started, but have trouble finishing them
Organized and will see a project through from start to finish
Slow at getting started, but good at getting things accomplished
34. Your friendships:
Change often and are made easily
Are mostly work-related or team-related
Last a very long time and are deeply meaningful

35. When it comes to money, you:
Like to shop and often overspend
Don't like to spend except on special items
Prefer not to spend and would rather save
36. Your dreams are:
Frequent and colorful
Romantic and occasional
Infrequent and disturbed, or intense

Determine Your Dosha

Sum up your answers to ascertain your dominant constitution. Your (A) answers are Vata, (B) Pitta, and (C) Kapha. The feature with the highest number of responses is the most prevalent in your overall constitution. Note, a dual dosha, like Vata-Pitta, Pitta-Kapha, or Vata-Kapha, is common. Although rarer, it is also possible to be equally balanced between all three.

Extra fat puts immense pressure on the heart, lungs, liver, and joints such as the thighs, knees, and ankles, making people overweight vulnerable to numerous diseases such as coronary thrombosis, high blood pressure, diabetes, arthritis, gout, liver, and gall bladder. Overeating, unhealthy eating habits are the primary cause of obesity and do not meet the laws of consuming or combining non-compatible food products in one meal.

Most western diets are focused on leaving out one of the essential food ingredients, such as sugar, protein, or carbohydrates. This type of deprived diet is not natural and health-dangerous. A healthy ayurvedic diet is promising for weight loss and weight retention. This Ayurvedic Diet fosters your strength and cleanses your body.

Ease your transformation into the diet with these pre-launch preparations before you start:

Take precautions: If you take medications, have had a medical operation recently, have a serious medical condition, or have any health concerns, have a look at the diet before you begin. Do not cleanse during pregnancy.

Eliminate dietary crutches: Eliminate all caffeinated and alcoholic beverages, dairy, meat, fried foods, processed foods, sugar, and any unhealthy meat you depend on during stressful times, for a few days or several weeks before the diet, so that giving them up does not become a shock to your system and psyche.

Take time off: The diet may be the way to spend a few days of your holiday and personal time before you lose them at the end of the year. To build the best diet environment, your days will be as stress-free as possible, with little to no work planned. According to Carlson, stress can cause digestive pain and constriction and prevent toxins from flowing out well from the body. "Taking the time to focus in a healthy lifestyle, self-care practices and yoga gives not only the chance to control and enhance physical digestion and removal but also provides the mind with a break from constant information 's intake, room for storing and digesting emotional and mental interactions and detoxifying the soul."

Build an area for home practice: If you do not have a designated practice room, place your yoga mats in your bedroom or living room, meditation pad, eye pillow, duvet, notebook, and inspirational books.

Unplug: Notify family and friends that you may be of social media and emails for some time. Unplugging social media and electronics decreases stress to the sense organs during the seasonal detox, and clears the memory.

Chapter 3: Week 1: Get started

The diet plan of 4 weeks contains eight components: meal, drink, five-sense purification, channel purification; seated meditation; eating; nature walks, and yoga.

Check the following calendar for an events plan for each of the four weeks, then use the detailed instructions as your toolkit. There are also some general guidelines: the plan is to provide three meals a day with minimal or zero snacks to make a break between meals in your digestive system. Eat each meal until you are satisfied and make your meal the lightest for lunch and dinner, so your body can process food before bed. And during meal breaks, perform health exercises that complement your diet, which is essential to a holistic detox approach.

Daily Routine

After waking up

Drink warm lemon water.

Complete the 5-senses purification.

Do channel-cleaning breathwork.

Meditate.

In the Morning

Eat breakfast. On weeks 1 and 4, eat only steamed vegetables and quinoa. On weeks 2 and 3, eat only simple kitchari.

Practice eating mindfully.

Walk-in nature.

Drink 1 cup of tea as desired.

In the Afternoon
Eat a large, satisfying lunch: Every day, lunch is a simple kitchari.
Practice mindful eating.
Sip 1 cup of tea as desired.
Avoid snacking. Alternatively, take warm water all day long. However, don't starve yourself if you're starving between meals. Snack on roasted almonds, which are easily digestible overnight.
Practice yoga for 20 to 60 minutes.
In the Evening
Take dinner: every day, dinner is harvest stew. Ensure to give yourself about 2–3 hours to digest this meal before bedtime.
Try to read books of inspiration, write a diary or meditate.
Go to bed early enough to sleep for 8 hours.
Mindful Eating
How you eat is just as important in Ayurveda as what you eat. If you eat when you are stressed or have a lot of work, or you don't focus on food, you can create indigestion because you don't chew thoroughly. Mindful eating helps promote healthy digestion so that you eat what you need of food for the mind and body and eliminate toxins. Tips for Mindful eating
Eat breakfast, lunch, and dinner every day around the same time to establish a digestive system routinely.
Enjoy a relaxing environment.
Minimize distractions and stimulation, for example, TV, computers, and mobile phones. You can listen and enjoy soothing music.

Eat meals in a comfortable and relaxed manner. Eat quietly or only take positive impressions. Avoid reading the crime news from the newspaper – instead, browse the arts section. Or better yet, take a glance out your window or take a look at the kitchen table with a flower.

Concentrate all conversation on positive topics when you eat with a company. Avoid debating, arguing, chattering, or complaining that may cause stress.

Take a few snacks before eating as you appreciate all the energy you gave to grow, harvest, transport, and prepare this beautiful meal.

Commit all your senses to the meal.

Appreciate colors, scenes, and scents. Chew slowly (take at least ten chews per bite). Taste the food's flavor and texture.

Take seconds into account. Meals can be on the bigger side to avoid snacking. However, stop for a few moments before you take another portion and see if your body wants more or not.

Take a few breaths at the end of each meal before you get up to feel the effects. Wait for a burp. Wait for a burp. When your stomach is full, the body gives you a natural burp. Notice that you are now satisfied, satisfied, and nourished by all your senses.

Chapter 4: Week 2: Detoxifying Drinks

To aid digestion during the diet, sip these beverages

1. Lemon water

Drink 1 cup of hot water with a fresh lemon squeeze that helps to remove excess mucus. Rehydration also helps with your bowel movement in the morning. Citrus adds flavor.

2. Teas

Pick one of the following cleaning teas, steep tea bag for up to 5 minutes in hot water, and drink an average of 2 cups a day. Enjoy the unique benefits of tea, noted by Drs in The Yoga of Herbs. Vasant Lad and David Frawley.

Tulsi (Holy Basil): Antiseptic, calming, and antibacterial characteristics of the tulsi help remove congestion from the lungs (for excess Kapha dosha) when soothing nerves (for excess Vata dosha).

Ginger: Ginger's expectorant, stimulant, and carminative effects help to remove extra phlegm and mucous in the body and to aid digestion.

Cumin-coriander-fennel: cumin improves digestion and absorption, coriander adds to the reduction of extra pitta and less inflammation, as well as fennel helps to reduce gasses while improving digestive energy.

Purification of the 5-Senses

Incorporate this morning self-care practice to aid the diet detoxification process.

Hearing: listen to nature, kirtan, and other calming music when you wake, to fill your ears with encouraging sounds. Say your family's loving words. And avoid the morning news.

See: Sprinkle the eyes with cold, filtered water 3–6 times after waking up in the morning to relax and loosen the eyes.

Taste: Use a tongue scraper to make 3 to 6 strong tongue scrapes to the tip from the back of the tongue, pulling away any white, yellow, or brown tongue particles, which are contaminants. Rinse your mouth and tongue scraper in between each scrape with filtered water. In a glass of moist, filtered water, dissolve 1/2 tsp of salt and gargle 3 to 6 times.

Smell: Dissolve 1/8 to 1/4 tsp of neti-pot salt in filtered hot water to remove your nose of bacteria and germs in a clean and purified neti-pot. Put half the solution through a sink and let it drain the other nose. On the other side, repeat. Blow your nose for extra mucus to be removed. Apply 1–2 drops of Nasya oil in each nostril (a blend of herbs like eucalyptus, calamus, and oil skullcap) to lubricate the nose cell and protect the mucous membranes.

Touch: Take an exfoliator (Darshana) massage on weeks 1 and 3 to prepare skin for oil absorbance in a daily massage with warm oil (abhyanga/snehana). Make light, long strokes on the long sides of your body with a dry loofah glove and circles at the joints for 1 to 2 minutes.

Before shower every day, perform a warm-oil massage to boost circulation, stimulate lymphatic system detoxification. Lube the skin up with a few tablespoons of warmed sesame oil. Pass over the entire body, stroke long on long bones, and arcs at the joints. Get into the shower and begin the wet massage, so the oil gets into your muscles. Then the soap areas which need to be washed (armpits, genitals, hands, feet), leaving the protective oil in place for others.

Chapter 5: Week 3: Yoga Series To Stoke Digestive Fire

This sequence is intended to stimulate the digestive fire with plenty of hips and abdominal work. Keep the breath deep and rhythmic to stimulate circulation during practice. Carlson recommends starting from 3 to 6 rounds of your favorite Sun Salutations variation if you want to extend your practice.

Breathwork for Channel Cleaning

Practice alternate Nadi shodhana breathing for 5 to 20 minutes a day before the meditation to relax the mind and ease the nervous system.

How to: Cover your right nose completely with your right thumb for one period and then softly inhale your left nose. Uncover your right nose and cover your right ring finger with your left hand. Exhale your right nose, then inhale your right nose. Uncover your left nose, cover your right nose with your right hand, and exhale your left nose. Have the breath be soft and rhythmic, repeat.

Take a walk in Nature.

Take a 15 to 30-minute daily walk through nature that increases harmony, balance, and peace and metabolism for detoxification.

How to: Try a nearby forest, park, garden, or waterfront — just how important it is to have an exact location and to avoid sensory stimulation (this is how to leave the earbuds at home!).

Seated meditation

Practice this sitting and hum meditation once or twice a day for 5 to 20 minutes, in the morning or evening, to anchor the concentration of the mind and encourage self-inquiry.

How to: sit on a chair, cushion, or meditation bench in a comfortable position. Remove hands to lap—longer from your tailbone to your head's crown. Close your eyes. Close your eyes. Relax the muscles of the nose. Smooth the back. Follow your breath. Follow your breath. On the inhaler, loop softly, and on the exhale, sigh. Let the mind concentrate on the mantra. Hum says, then, "I am that," you are telling yourself, "What am I?" As the mind walks, lead it gently back to the mantra center, accompanying the wind. Upon completion, release the mantra and take a few breaths to feel the experience and to note whether your mind is more spacious and clear.

Chapter 6: Week 4: After the diet

It may be enticing to go for pizza and beer when you end wrap up your diet routine. But that could shake the body and cancel all of your dedicated work more quickly than you can tell, "Extra cheese, please." The detox process continues for days after you finish the diet so you can move easily into your normal diet. Follow these tips for the remainder of the days to bond completely into your body and achieve lasting benefits.

Eat foods that are cooked. They are easier to digest, especially during the late fall Vata season. Avoid heavy and dense foods requiring more digestive energy, such as red meat, hard cheeses, and pasta.

Drink warm lemon water for hydration in the morning. Dehydration is marked by thirst, dry lips or eyes, and constipation.

Every night, get at least eight hours of sleep.

Get back to your usual practice or yoga routine gradually.

Eat mindfully.

Recipes you can try
To aid your stimulation, we have put together some easy to prepare Ayurvedic Recipes that you can try while on your diet lifestyle.

Kitchari

Ingredients:

1 cup basmati rice

½ cup yellow mung dal

1 tablespoon Kitchari Spice Mix*

2 tablespoons ghee

6 cups of water

1–2 cups chopped vegetables (optional)

Optional garnishes and spice additions:

Fresh cilantro (great for pitta—ok for vata and kapha)

Coconut (great for pitta, good for vata, but not so good for kapha)

Lime (ok for everybody)

Salt to taste (optional).

Directions:

Wash rice and mung dal and soak overnight. Drain soak water.

In a medium saucepan warm the ghee. Add the Kitchari Spice Mix and sauté for one to two minutes. Add rice and mung dal and sauté for another couple of minutes. Then add 6 cups of water and bring to a boil.

Once the kitchari has come to a boil reduce the heat to medium-low. Cover and cook until it is tender (approx. 30–45 minutes).

If you are adding vegetables to your kitchari, add the longer cooking vegetables, such as carrots and beets, halfway through the cooking. Add the vegetables that cook faster, such as leafy greens, near the end.

Add more water if needed. Typically, kitchari is the consistency of a vegetable stew as opposed to a broth. A thinner consistency is preferable if your digestion is weak. You will notice that kitchari will thicken when it cools and you may need more water than you originally thought.

Detox Bowl

Ingredients

½ C diced onion

1 ½ T olive oil or coconut oil

1 T grated ginger

1 T chopped garlic

1 tsp whole mustard seeds

1 tsp turmeric

½ tsp cumin

½ tsp coriander

1/2 tsp curry powder, more to taste

1 small dried red chili pepper, crumbled(or half for less spicy)

¾ tsp kosher salt

¼ cup split mung beans, split lentils (or whole mung beans or whole lentils- soaked overnight)

½ cup toasted buckwheat (Kashi) or (soaked, brown basmati rice)

1 ½ cup water

1 cup veggie broth

2 Cups chopped vegetables (like carrot, parsnips, celery, a fennel bulb, cauliflower, broccoli)

2 tablespoon chopped cilantro or Italian parsley

Squeeze lemon or lime

1 diced tomato

Instructions

In a medium pot, saute onion in oil over medium-high heat for 2-3 minutes. Reduce heat to medium add ginger and garlic, and saute a few minutes, until golden and fragrant.

Add spices, pepper, and salt and stir, toast for a few more minutes. Add soaked mung beans and buckwheat or soaked brown rice. Add water, broth and 2 cups chopped veggies bring to a good boil. Cover. Turn heat to low, and let simmer for 20 minutes. Check for doneness.

Continue cooking for 5 to 10 more minutes if necessary. Some rice takes longer, and if you do not pre-soak your whole mung beans or brown rice, you will need to add more water, which will change the recipe proportions and flavor...so try to soak if possible.

Once it is done, taste and adjust salt and seasonings. If you like a more "porridge-like" consistency add more veggie broth.

Spoon into bowls, top with fresh diced tomato and fresh cilantro or parsley and a pinch of salt and pepper, and a squeeze of lemon or lime.

A drizzle a little olive oil over the top of the tomatoes is nice too.

Masala Rice

Ingredients
2 cups basmati rice
1/2 cup zucchini, chopped
1/2 cup green beans, chopped1/2 cup fresh peas
(carrots, potatoes, cauliflower, or broccoli may
be substituted according to the constitution)
1/2 tsp cumin seeds
1/2 tsp black mustard seeds
1/4 tsp turmeric
1 pinch asafoetida (hing)
2 pinches salt
12 – 14 cloves, whole1-inch piece of fresh ginger,
peeled and diced fine
2 cinnamon sticks, broken into small pieces
6 – 10 bay leaves
10 cardamom pods, whole
1 pinch cayenne
3 cloves garlic, chopped fine
1/2 cup ghee
1 Tbs coconut, shredded
1/2 cup cilantro, fresh, chopped (divided use)
1 lime

Preparation
Wash the rice two times. Wash and chop vegetables.
Put the chopped ginger and ¼ cup of the cilantro in a blender with coconut and ½ cup of water. Blend until liquid.

Heat the ghee in a 3-quart saucepan and add the mustard seeds, cumin seeds, turmeric, and hing, and cook until the mustard seeds pop. Then add the cloves, bay leaves, cardamom, and cinnamon. Heat until the spices are fragrant then pour in the blended mixture. Add the garlic and salt, and then cook until the garlic browns slightly. Stir in the vegetables and rice, mixing thoroughly. Add cayenne. Pour in 5 cups of water and bring to a boil. Turn down the heat to a simmer and cover loosely.

Cook until the vegetables are tender and the rice is cooked for about 18 to 20 minutes. Turn this out into a serving dish and squeeze fresh lime juice over it. Sprinkle chopped cilantro and coconut over the top before serving.

Mediterranean Salad

Ingredients
3 – 4 cups leafy greens of your choice
Avocado dressing
1 cup lentil-zucchini mix
1 cup couscous
1 cup beets
6 Tbs. soft goat cheese
Fresh ground black pepper
Cilantro, fresh, chopped fine

Preparation
Toss the greens with the avocado dressing and arrange on serving plate or bowl. Then layer the lentils, couscous, and beets (see recipes below) on top of the dressed greens. Drop the goat cheese by tablespoons around the platter. Grind a bit of pepper on top and sprinkle with chopped cilantro.

Lentil-Veggie Marinade

Simmer together for 20 minutes: 1 cup water, 1/4 cup French lentils, and 1 pinch of hing. While this is cooking, mix 1/4 cup fennel, chopped, and 2 Tbs. dill with a pinch of salt and pepper, 1 Tbs. rice vinegar, and 2 tsp. olive oil. Lightly sauté 1/2 cup zucchini in chopped shallots, sunflower oil, and rice vinegar. Cool the lentils and zucchini then mix all ingredients together and let marinate in the refrigerator overnight or for 4 hours.

Couscous

Sauté 1/2 cup Israeli (pearl) couscous with 2 tsp. sunflower oil for 2 – 3 minutes. Add 3/4 cup water or broth, bring to a boil then reduce heat to simmer 10 – 15 minutes. Toss together with 2 Tbs. chopped parsley, juice of 1/2 lemon, 1/2 tsp. salt, and 1/4 tsp. pepper. Can use warm or prepare ahead and refrigerate.

Cooking the Beets

Take one medium to large-sized red or golden beet and cut in quarters. Peel the tough outer layer away. Steam the quarters in a covered pan with a steamer basket and 1 inch of water for 20 minutes, until done. Allow to cool, chop into 1/2 inch pieces, and store in the refrigerator until ready to assemble the salad.

Avocado dressing

1 small ripe avocado
1 Tbs. lime juice
2 Tbs. rice vinegar
1/2 cup olive oil
1 tablespoon chopped parsley
1 tablespoon chopped cilantro
Salt and pepper to taste
Cut the avocado in half, working around the pit.
Twist apart and remove the pit with a knife.
Scoop out the flesh with a teaspoon and put it in
a blender or small food processor. Add the
remaining ingredients and blend until smooth
and well mixed then season with salt and fresh
ground pepper.

Red Cabbage Salad

Ingredients

1 small red cabbage, sliced thin
1 sweet banana pepper, chopped
1/4 cup sweet onion, chopped (optional)
1 small beet, grated
1 carrot, grated
1 baby zucchini, chopped
1/4 cup roasted sunflower seeds
A few sprigs of fresh parsley

Salad Dressing

1/3 cup olive oil
1 Tablespoon lemon juice
1 Tablespoon honey
1 teaspoon Dijon mustard
Salt and pepper to taste

Preparation

Combine all veggies in a large bowl.

Whisk together dressing ingredients and pour over veggies. Serve with warm chapatti or tortilla.

The sweetness of this salad will pacify hot pitta, the oil in the dressing should address vata and the honey will help pacify Kapha.

Ayurvedic Oatmeal
Ingredients
200 ml of water
200 g (1 cup) pumpkin flesh, cut in small cubes
1-2 tbsp raisins
80 g oatmeal flakes
300 ml soy or any other vegan milk
2 cinnamon sticks
1/4 tsp ground cardamon and/or 1/8 tsp ground cloves
2 cm of turmeric (Curcuma) root, peeled and rasped, or 1/2 tsp ground turmeric
1-2 tbsp pumpkin seeds or to taste
Preparation
Cover the pumpkin cubes and raisins with water and bring to boil. Cook on low heat for ten minutes.
Add soy (or any other vegan) milk and bring it to boil again.
Add oatmeal flakes, cinnamon sticks, cardamom powder, and turmeric. Cook for another ten minutes.
Sprinkle with the pumpkin seeds and serve.

Conclusion

Thank you again for getting this guide.

If you found this guide helpful, please take the time to share your thoughts and post a review. It'd be greatly appreciated!

Thank you and good luck!

Printed in Great Britain
by Amazon

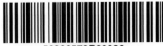
56866579R20026